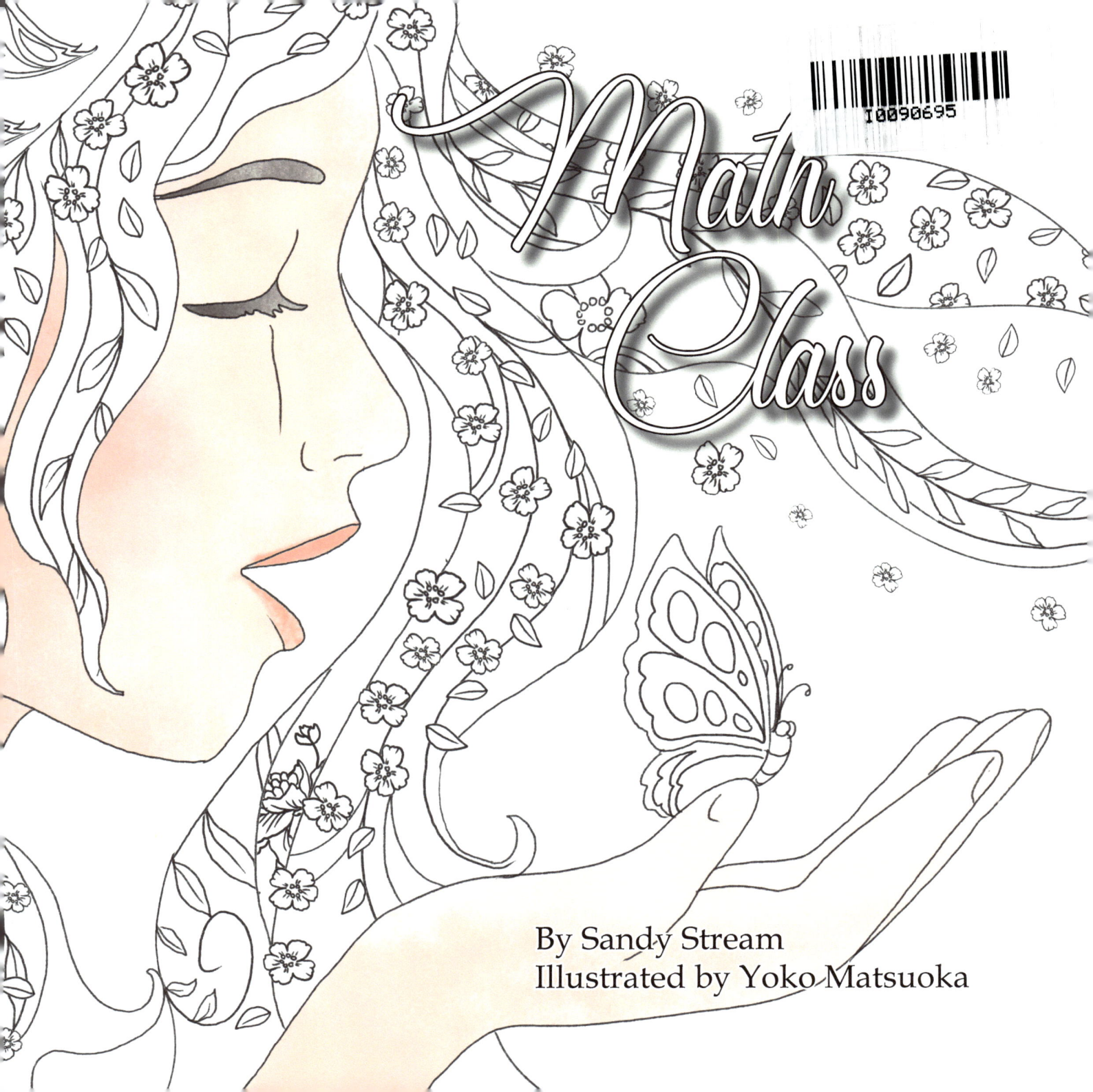

Math Class

By Sandy Stream

Illustrated by Yoko Matsuoka

Math Class. By Sandy Stream
Illustrated by Yoko Matsuoka
Edited by Tomoko Matsuoka
ISBN: 978-0-9938828-3-8

Sensitivity

What does it mean to be sensitive? To feel what is happening around you? To feel what other people feel? What you feel?

Many people might want to reduce their sensitivity, having been told that it's not a good thing. That you need to toughen up to make it through life.

But is it better to go through life that way — not feeling? Being numb to what is actually happening? Is that really being alive? Or is one more alive by being sensitive, even if it means experiencing some pain?

What would you choose? A life being sensitive, which will include feeling some pain, or a long life of being insensitive?

I have made my choice.

Sandy Stream

The Garden

There was once a little girl with no name. The little girl lived in a town where each person had a garden of their own. And in every garden, lived a wise fairy that took care of the garden.

The little girl visited the garden every day and brought food to the wise fairy. The wise fairy smiled and calmly distributed the food to the different plants and bugs in the garden.

The garden had many little creatures in it. It had Builders who liked to build, and Breakers who broke things, but they all lived in harmony. The wise fairy was careful not to give too much food to the Breakers, making sure everything stayed in balance.

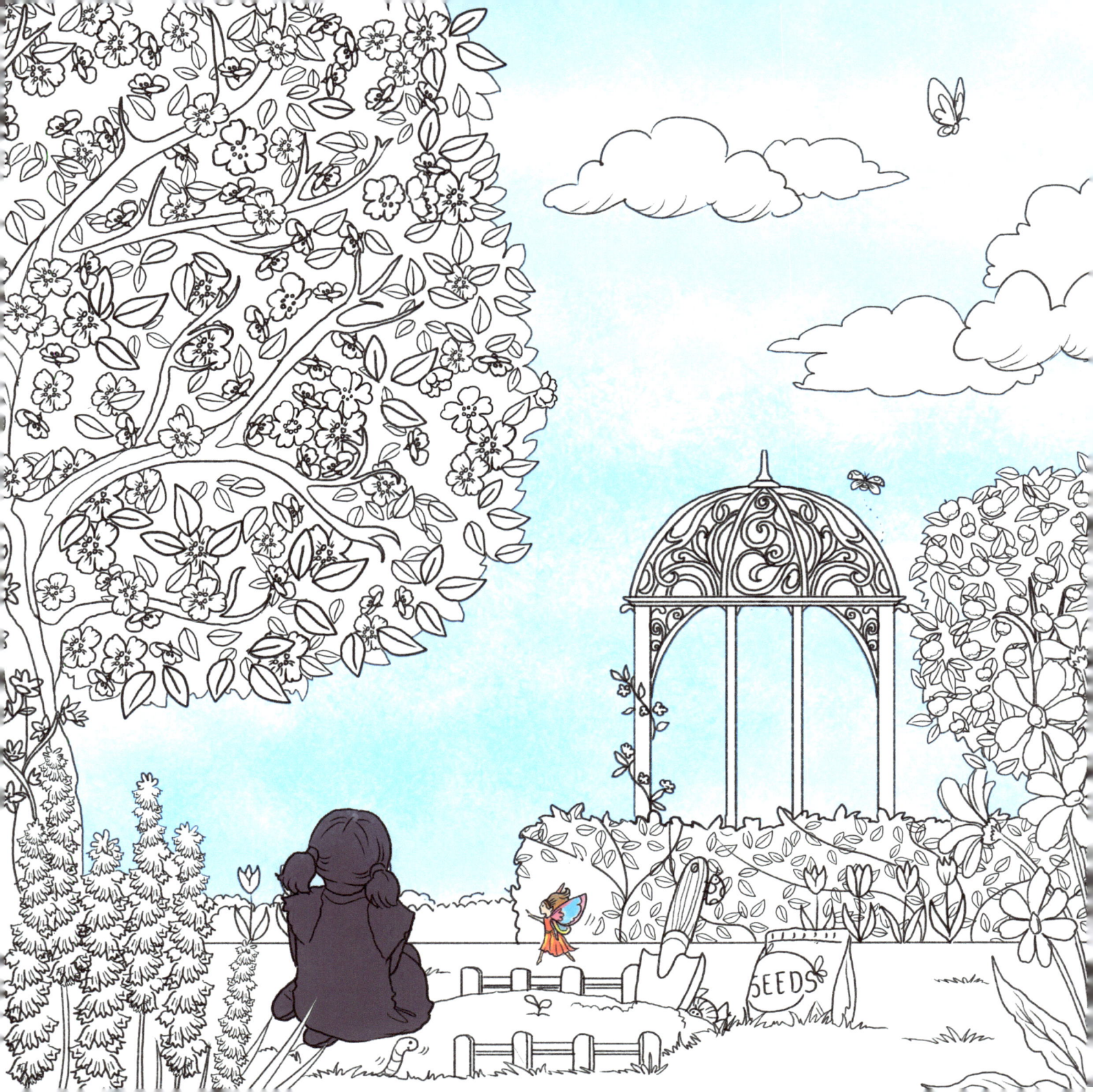

The little girl with no name didn't know much about gardening. She sometimes threw garbage into the garden without realizing what it did.

The Breakers began to multiply and the wise fairy became upset. She was not able to keep the garden clean and balanced anymore. She tried to speak to the girl, but the girl would not listen. Whenever the girl approached the garden to put things in it, the fairy became very nervous. But the girl still did not listen.

Years passed, and the girl with no name got older and became a young woman with no name. The garden smelled fowl and the Breakers in the garden multiplied and grew stronger. The wise fairy was no longer able to control them. They started breaking through the fence surrounding the garden and invaded the young woman's home, and she became sick.

Then one day, the wise fairy spoke to the young woman and asked for help. "Please," she said, "will you help me mend the garden?" The young woman with no name opened her eyes and finally understood. She needed to take care of her garden. And so began the woman's journey of looking inside and listening to the fairy.

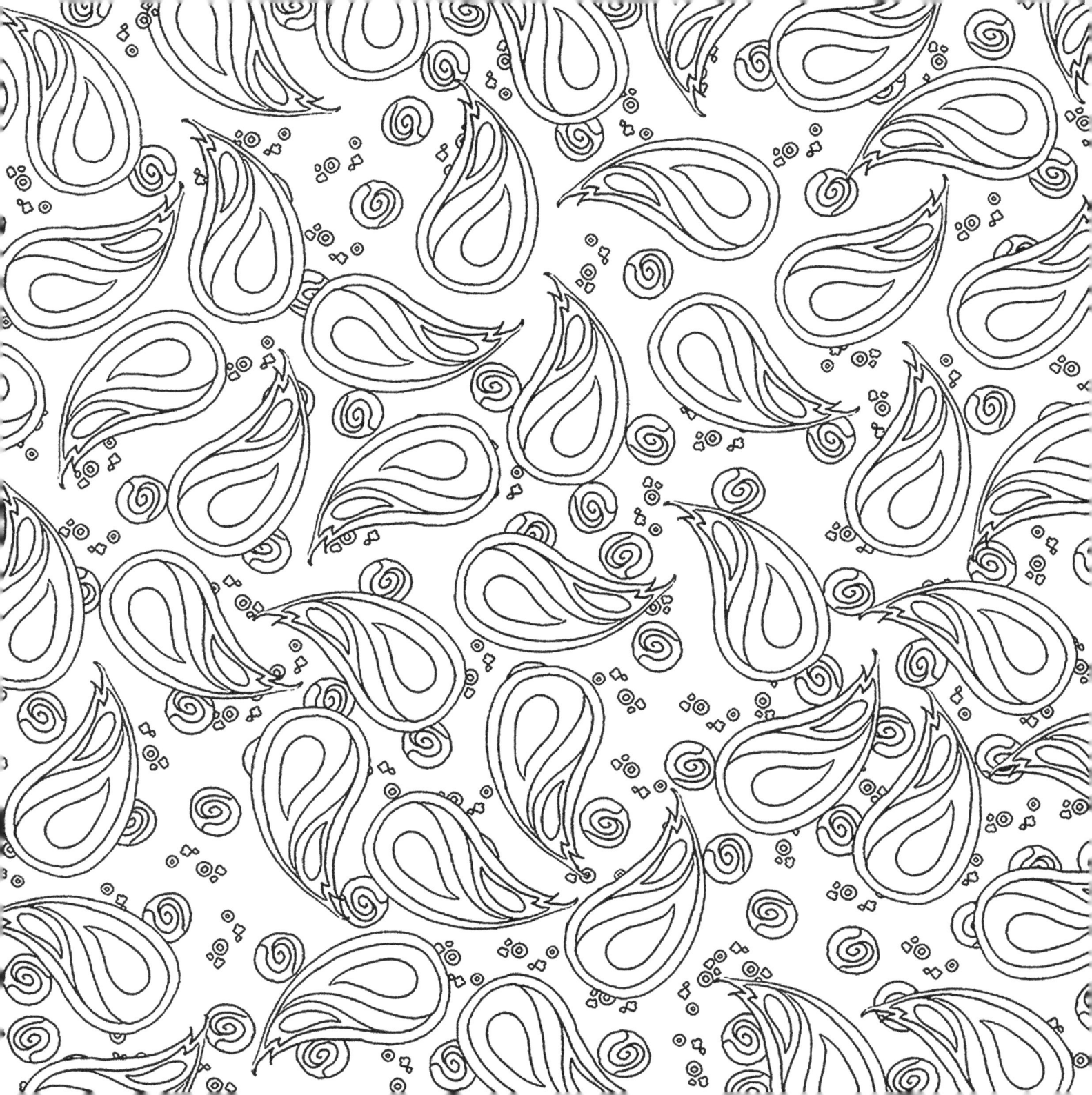

THE PATH TO HEALING

The woman with no name began walking on the path to healing and on this path, she saw two signs. One sign said **"Math School"** and the other sign said **"Healing Field."** She chose the road to the **"Healing Field"** and continued walking.

At the end of the path there was a beautiful field. She figured that this is where she would heal. But as she spent time in the field, she felt even worse!

The earth that she thought would help her get grounded really hurt her feet. The hot sun, which she was told would give her energy, made her weaker. The wind was cold and made her shiver.

Even the water from the nearby river and the berries from the bushes didn't help. Her garden inside felt even worse…

She saw an old man sitting under a tree. He walked slowly and gently towards her and asked her how she felt in the healing field.

"I thought the field would give me everything I need, but it didn't help me," she said desperately.

"You have to fix your math first before coming here," he said. "Go back to the sign where you saw 'Math School' and follow that path before you come here, to the healing field."

She didn't understand why, since she thought she was quite adept at math, but she went anyway.

MaTH CLASS

She followed the sign to the math school and arrived at an opening in the forest. Many children were sitting facing a beautiful teacher. The young woman with no name felt herself shrinking and becoming a little child again. She took little steps and joined the class and sat with all the other children.

"Good morning, students," said the lovely teacher. "I know you might feel uncomfortable being here. This class can be hard — very hard, sometimes.

"Today we will learn math — or, actually, we will unlearn your *bad math*."

No one said anything.

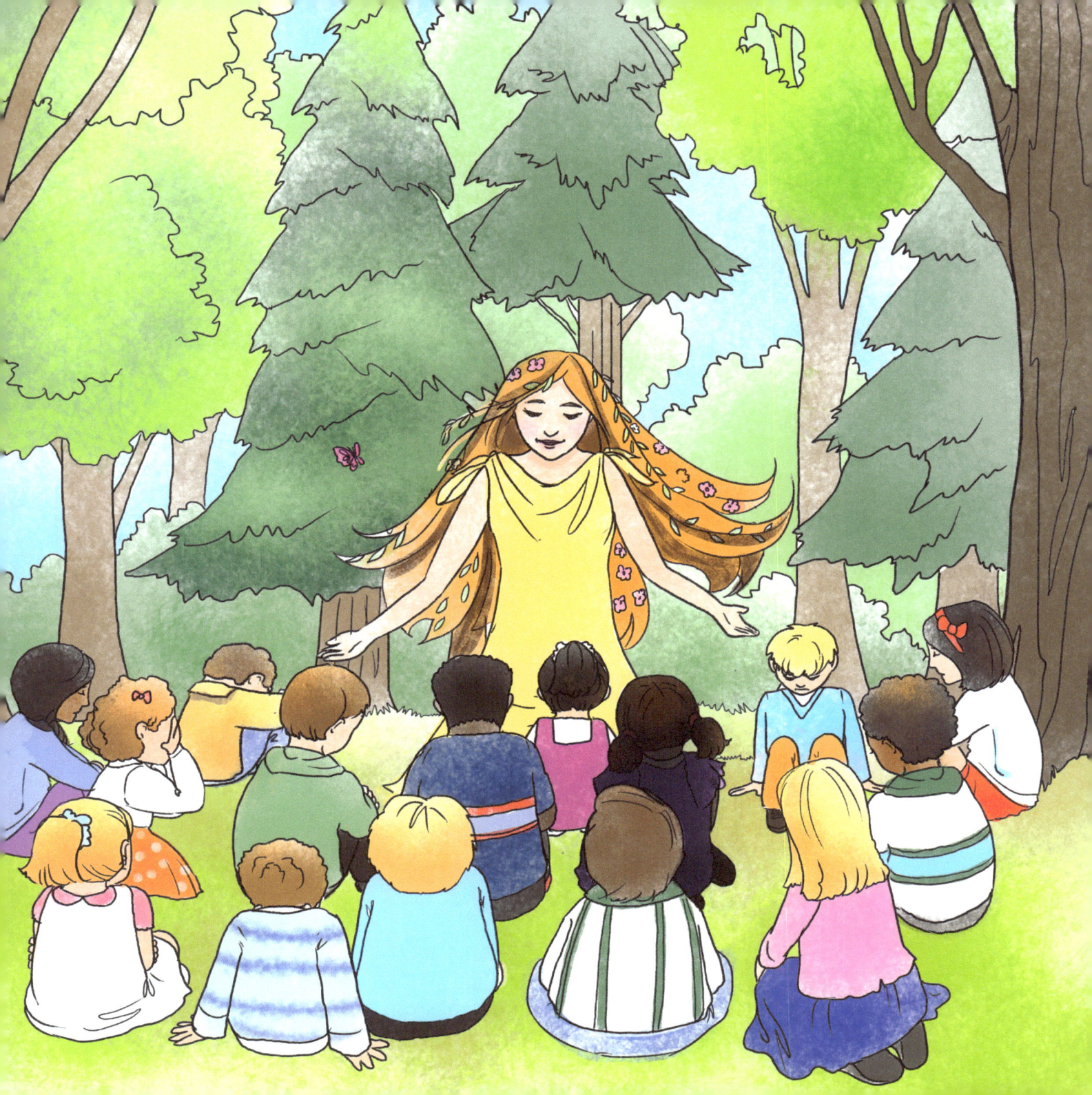

"Let us begin," the teacher said. "When you were young, you were taught two math equations:

1. If you are GOOD, you will get good things, rewards. If GOOD => get GOOD

2. If you are BAD, you will get punishment or something negative.

   If BAD => get BAD

The whole class nodded.

"Well," said the teacher smiling, "this is why you are here. You all believe these equations, but they are wrong. We will fix your bad math."

"Has anyone ever gotten something negative from life, from parents, or from your friends? Have you been yelled at? Put down? Unloved? Ignored? Anything negative?" the teacher asked gently.

Everyone nodded.

"When you did not get good things, you assumed that something in you was not good, not quite right. When you got bad things, a part of you did some bad math and assumed you must be bad. This is why you are here.

"If there is even a tiny part of you that believes this to be true, we must fix your bad math. Even the healing field cannot help if you do not believe that you deserve good things.

"So let's sit quietly now for 30 minutes and ask our bodies and minds honestly…. Is there even a little part of you that that thinks you are bad? Not good enough? Not normal? Not deserving? That you did something unforgivable?

"If there a part of you that believes that your truest self is not good enough, then it's time to correct and fix your bad math."

No one believed anything the teacher said…

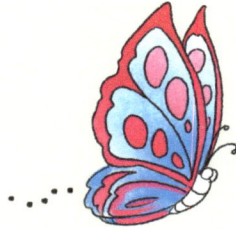

Then, after a long silence, one student spoke softly…

Student 1: "But I didn't do anything to help my sister get away."

Teacher: "That was not you, it was your fear. You wanted to help."

Student 2: "My dad got very angry at me… I must have deserved it somehow. I am no good."

Teacher: "This is bad math. You did not deserve that anger. You did not deserve bad things. You deserve only good things."

Student 3: "I am so mad about what my parents did. They deserve to be punished. I am a bad person for thinking this, but I can't help it."

Teacher: "Your body feels this because your body didn't have the chance to defend itself. Let your body feel the anger and imagine defending itself and then your body will feel better."

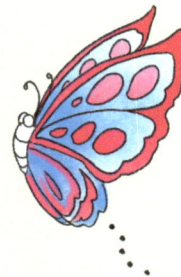

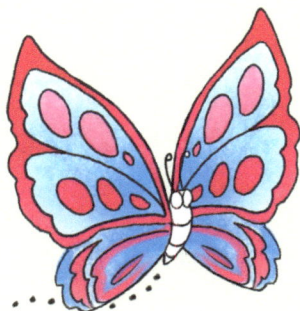

Student 4: "I didn't get hugs or love from my parents. There must be something wrong with me."

Teacher: "You went to your parent as any child does. But they did not pick you up. Your parent did not see your light inside. This has nothing to do with you. You should keep shining as you were meant to shine."

Student 5: "But I let him do it. I didn't stop him. I even liked it at first."

Teacher: "You were too frozen, too confused, and too young to do anything. Understand and forgive yourself. You are good."

Student 6: "I should not have dressed that way."

Teacher: "What happened was not your fault. You did not deserve what happened. You got bad things, but this does not mean you are bad! If a butterfly gets injured, does that make it bad? Does that make her unbeautiful?"

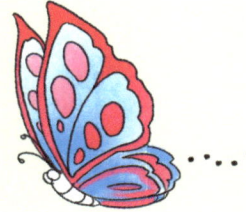

Student 7: "But I didn't tell anyone."

Teacher: "Your voice was closed. Use your voice now to express yourself fully."

Student 8: "I couldn't do anything. I have no power. I am nothing."

Teacher: "You have a lot of power. Start to use it."

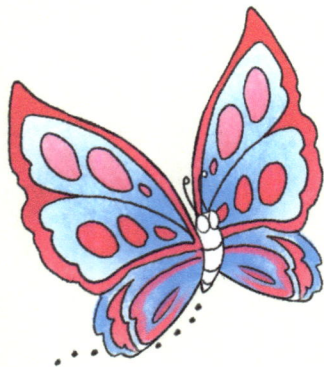

Student 9: "But I didn't follow god's rules."

Teacher: "Follow yourself and the Truth within you and know that you deserve all good things."

Student 10: "I know I had good reason to do what I did, but I still did it and I can't get over it."

Teacher: "Your mind understands what you did, but your body still feels bad for what it did. Forgive yourself for what you did — then you will no longer be against yourself. And you can start to feel the sun."

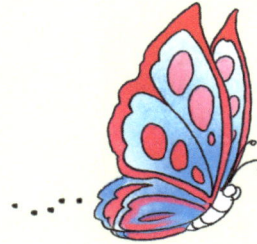

Student 11: "I didn't exist."

Teacher: "You did not exist in their eyes. But you do exist in reality. Exist and shine."

Student 12: "I could not live up to what they wanted me to do and be."

Teacher: "You are you. Just be yourself, not who others want you to be. Do not close up or huddle. Express yourself."

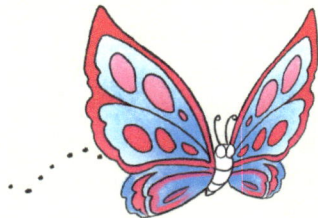

Student 13: "But I shouldn't feel this way. They tried."

Teacher: "This is not about how you should feel, it's about how you do feel. Just look at the truth of what your feelings are. Just look at them and let them be.

Student 14: "But I did bad things."

Teacher: "You did things because you didn't understand how to deal with pain. Your body did not know how to deal with your anguish in a different way. Forgive yourself and teach others so that your suffering has a good purpose."

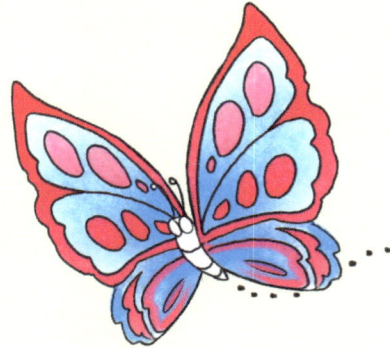

Student 15: "They used me and treated me like an object. They didn't treat me like a person. I am not a person."

Teacher: "I see you. All of you. You belong in this world."

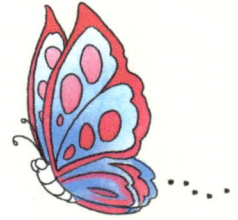

And the reader of this book said:

"_____
_____
_____
_____"

And the teacher said:

"_____
_____
_____
_____"

And the girl with no name said: "I was not allowed to be myself."

And the teacher said, looking right into the girl's soul:

"This is true and how hard that must have been. Come out now and you will blossom."

"SO WHY?!" cried all the kids.

"If we deserved everything good, why did they get so upset? Why didn't they love us? Why did all this happen?"

All the children were angry for weeks, recalling how they were treated, how they felt.

The teacher let them be upset for 30 days.

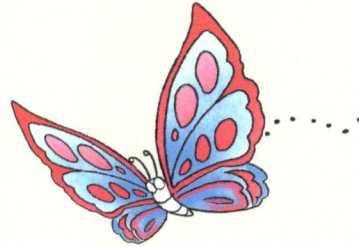

Then she softly whispered into their hearts…

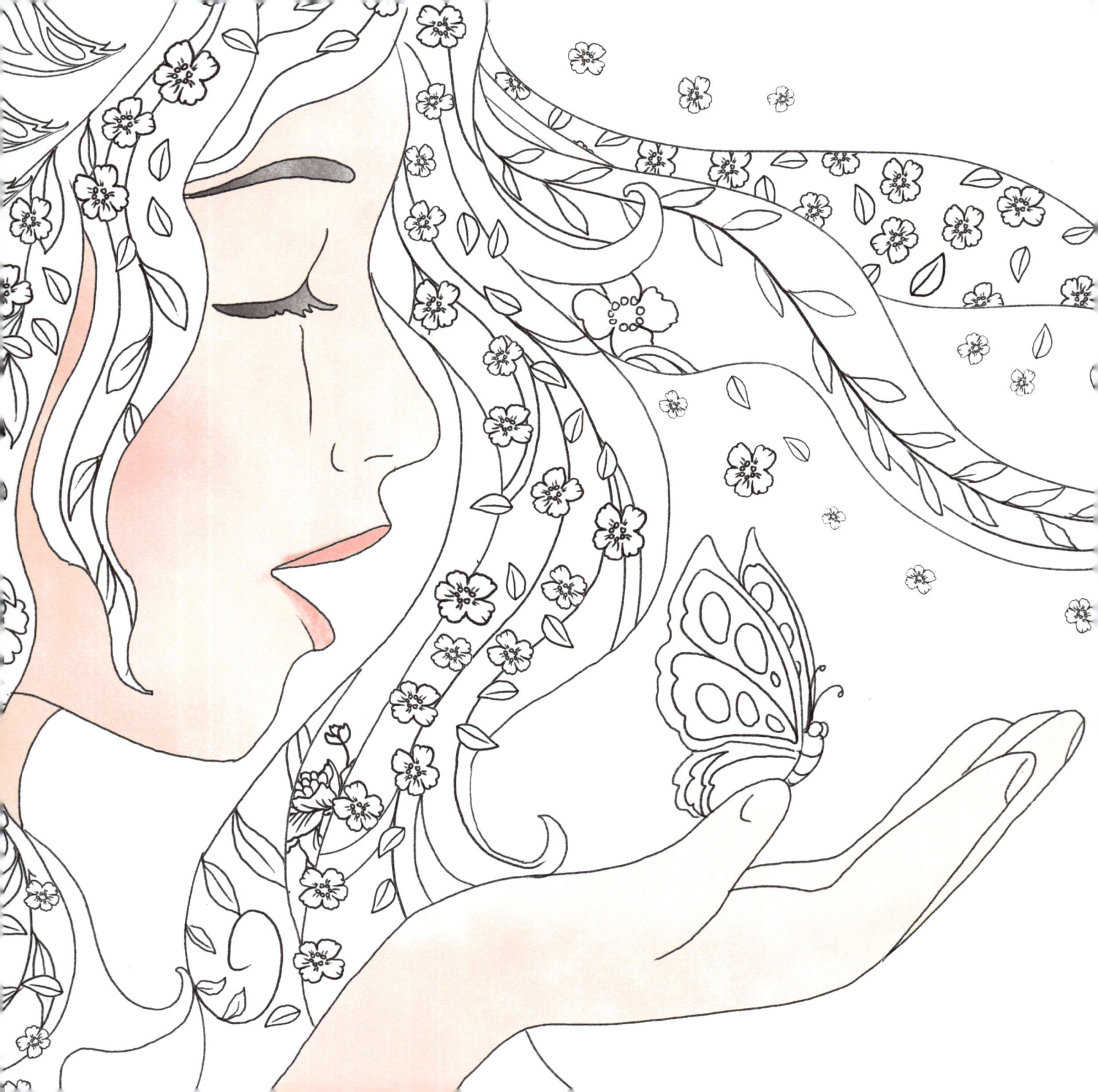

"It had nothing to do with you, my children…

It had nothing to do with you."

"Now it's time for you to shine. Do not be closed, huddled, not expressing your true self. You did not deserve the negative. You deserved all good things. You belong in this world."

All the children cried and then they finally lay down and could rest and sleep deeply and peacefully. "It had nothing to do with me," each said as they slid into their dreams…

When they woke up, they were ready to do the math test.

Everyone had to take the math test. "You must get 100% on this exam to pass," said the teacher. "If you answer false to even one question, you will need to redo this math class until you fix your math."

MATH TEST

Even if bad things happened to me, I did not deserve them	true false
Even if I didn't get good, I am good and deserve good	true false
I will allow myself to be my true self	true false
Even if I wasn't accepted, I accept myself	true false
Even if I didn't get the love I needed, I love myself	true false
My body believes I deserve health and happiness	true false
I will not punish myself in any way	true false
I will express myself fully and honestly	true false
It had nothing to do with me	true false

When the girl with no name finished the class and passed the math exam, she became grown up again and was ready to leave. She now knew that she had deserved good things and still does, thanks to her math teacher.

The Healing Field

The girl with no name walked to the healing field. She stood and opened her crown and let the energy in from the skies above. She pressed her feet on the earth and felt the ground underneath, and it gave her more energy. The sun faced her and she opened her skin and absorbed what it needed to revive her.

The wind blew gentle, cold air. She opened her eyes and felt it refresh her, reviving her system and softly urging her to move.

She opened her lips and drank the water.

She felt the waves from the distant ocean and breathed in the air of the ocean waves, which began softening her inside. The waves became more and more steady. She felt ready to go home and tend to her garden.

She went back home and started taking care of her garden.

She looked at her belly and saw how many things she was holding there; the many memories about all the moments and experiences, all formed knots in her belly. It was time to let these past experiences go. She sat on the ground and let the energy seep into the ground. She let the knots unravel.

She started feeding her garden very slowly, listening to its every request and movement, starting with warm soup for feeding the Builders. The Builders started building a new wall for her and became stronger than the Breakers again. She learned to trust herself, even though no one had ever trusted her before. She learned to trust her fairy for she knew better than anyone how to take care of the garden. It took a long time and a lot of courage.

Then she lay down to rest. She felt her navel, how she had shut it for so long not allowing anything in. She opened her navel, let all the energies in, good and bad, and they went through her and into the ground.

Her navel remained open from that day and began receiving light.

As she uncurled from her rounded position, she began discovering herself… until the light inside her literally popped open from its folded space… into a flower.

And slowly this flower began to blossom.

And on this day, she decided to give herself a name: *Jasmine.*

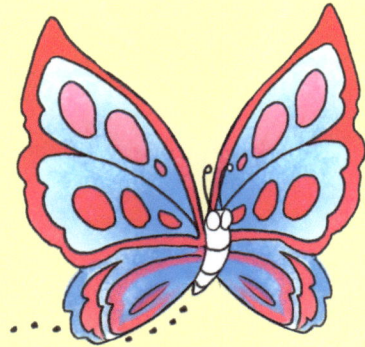

The beginning…

www.ingramcontent.com/pod-product-compliance
Lightning Source LLC
Chambersburg PA
CBHW041240020426
42333CB00002B/34